THE OPTIMAL STAGE 3 KIDNEY DISEASE DIET COOKBOOK FOR SENIORS

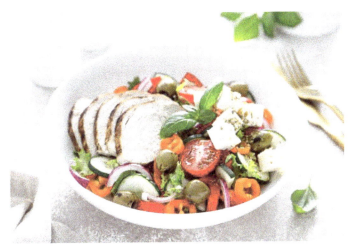

A Complete Guide To A Healthy and Delicious Diet, Meal Plans, Diet/Lifestyle Tips and Juicing Recipes

THE KITCHEN SAGE

Copyright © 2023 by THE KITCHEN SAGE

All rights reserved. No part of this book may be reproduced, distributed, or transmitted in any form or by any means, including photocopying, recording, or other electronic or mechanical methods, without the prior written permission of the author, except in the case of brief quotations embodied in critical reviews and certain other non-commercial uses permitted by copyright law.
For permissions requests or inquiries, please contact
First Edition
2023
All rights reserved.

TABLE OF CONTENT

INTRODUCTION 9

Chapter 1: KIDNEY DISEASE DIET BASICS 11

    What is Kidney Disease and Stage 3 Kidney Disease? 11

    How Does Diet Affect Kidney Disease? 12

    The Importance of Eating Well with Kidney Disease 12

    What to Expect in This Book 13

CHAPTER 2: What Nutrients are Important for People with Kidney Disease? 14

    What Nutrients Should Be Limited? 15

    How to Read Food Labels 15

    Tips for Cooking Kidney-Friendly Meals 16

DELICIOUS BREAKFAST RECIPES 17

    Recipe 1: Creamy Oatmeal with Berries 17

    Recipe 2: Greek Yogurt Parfait 17

    Recipe 3: Scrambled Egg Whites with Spinach and Tomatoes 18

    Recipe 4: Cottage Cheese Pancakes 18

    Recipe 5: Spinach and Feta Omelette 19

    Recipe 6: Whole Grain Toast with Avocado and Poached Egg 19

    Recipe 7: Apple Cinnamon Quinoa Bowl 20

    Recipe 8: Sweet Potato and Spinach Hash 20

    Recipe 9: Chia Seed Pudding with Almonds and Berries ... 21

Recipe 10: Muesli with Greek Yogurt and Honey _____ 21

Recipe 11: Almond Butter and Banana Wrap _____ 22

Recipe 12: Berry Blast Smoothie _____ 22

Recipe 13: Spinach and Feta Breakfast Burrito _____ 23

Recipe 14: Banana Nut Overnight Oats _____ 23

Recipe 15: Veggie and Cheese Omelette _____ 24

Recipe 16: Cinnamon Raisin Toast with Cottage Cheese ___ 24

Recipe 17: Pineapple and Cottage Cheese Bowl _____ 25

Recipe 18: Avocado and Tomato Toast with Poached Egg __ 25

Recipe 19: Blueberry Almond Smoothie Bowl _____ 26

Recipe 20: Spinach and Mushroom Frittata _____ 26

EASY AND DELICIOUS LUNCH RECIPES _____ *28*

Recipe 1: Grilled Salmon Salad _____ 28

Recipe 2: Quinoa and Vegetable Stir-Fry _____ 28

Recipe 3: Turkey and Avocado Wrap _____ 29

Recipe 4: Spinach and Chickpea Salad _____ 29

Recipe 5: Egg Salad Lettuce Wraps _____ 30

Recipe 6: Lentil and Vegetable Soup _____ 30

Recipe 7: Tuna and White Bean Salad _____ 30

Recipe 8: Caprese Salad with Balsamic Glaze _____ 31

Recipe 9: Chicken and Vegetable Skewers _____ 31

Recipe 10: Greek Yogurt Chicken Salad _____ 32

Recipe 11: Sweet Potato and Black Bean Bowl _____ 32

Recipe 12: Spinach and Goat Cheese Stuffed Chicken Breast 33

Recipe 13: Cauliflower and Broccoli Soup _____ 33

Recipe 14: Shrimp and Asparagus Stir-Fry _____ 34

Recipe 15: Chickpea and Avocado Salad _____ 34

Recipe 16: Broccoli and Cheddar Stuffed Sweet Potato ____ 35

Recipe 17: Turkey and Spinach Wrap with Hummus _____ 35

Recipe 18: Tomato Basil Mozzarella Salad _____ 36

Recipe 19: Tofu and Vegetable Stir-Fry _____ 36

Recipe 20: Spinach and Feta Stuffed Chicken Breast_____ 37

QUICK AND EASY DINNER RECIPES _____ *38*

Recipe 1: Baked Lemon Herb Salmon _____ 38

Recipe 2: Spinach and Tomato Stuffed Bell Peppers _____ 38

Recipe 3: Turkey and Vegetable Stir-Fry _____ 39

Recipe 4: Cauliflower Rice with Shrimp and Peas _____ 39

Recipe 5: Eggplant and Tomato Caprese _____ 40

Recipe 6: Chicken and Vegetable Skillet _____ 41

Recipe 7: Stuffed Portobello Mushrooms _____ 41

Recipe 8: Beef and Broccoli Stir-Fry _____ 42

Recipe 9: Zucchini Noodles with Pesto and Cherry Tomatoes _____ 42

Recipe 10: Greek Chicken and Vegetable Skewers _____ 43

Recipe 11: Lentil and Spinach Curry_____ 43

Recipe 12: Baked Chicken Thighs with Herbs _____ 44

Recipe 13: Tomato and Spinach Frittata _____ 44

Recipe 14: Tofu and Vegetable Curry_____ 45

Recipe 15: Spaghetti Squash with Tomato Sauce _____ 45

Recipe 16: Shrimp and Asparagus Bake _____ 46

Recipe 17: Spinach and Feta Stuffed Turkey Burger _____ 46

Recipe 18: Broccoli and Cheddar Stuffed Chicken Thigh ___ 47

Recipe 19: Caprese Stuffed Portobello Mushrooms _____ 47

Recipe 20: Pesto Zucchini Noodles with Grilled Chicken ___ 48

DELICIOUS SNACKS AND DESSERT RECIPES _____ 49

Recipe 1: Cucumber and Hummus Bites _____ 49

Recipe 2: Greek Yogurt with Berries _____ 49

Recipe 3: Almonds and Dried Apricots _____ 50

Recipe 4: Cottage Cheese with Pineapple _____ 50

Recipe 5: Baked Sweet Potato Fries _____ 50

Recipe 6: Hard-Boiled Eggs with Paprika _____ 51

Recipe 7: Rice Cake with Almond Butter and Banana _____ 51

Recipe 8: Carrot Sticks with Hummus _____ 52

Recipe 9: Berry Parfait _____ 52

Recipe 10: Baked Apple with Cinnamon _____ 52

Recipe 11: Chia Seed Pudding with Almonds and Berries __ 53

Recipe 12: Banana and Walnut Muffins _____ 53

Recipe 13: Dark Chocolate Covered Strawberries _____ 54

Recipe 14: Vanilla Yogurt with Sliced Almonds _____ 54

Recipe 15: Peach and Cottage Cheese Bowl _____ 55

Recipe 16: Oatmeal Raisin Cookies _____ 55

Recipe 17: Baked Pears with Cinnamon _____ 56

Recipe 18: Blueberry Yogurt Parfait _____ 56

Recipe 19: Chocolate Banana Smoothie_____ 56

Recipe 20: Apple and Cinnamon Rice Cake _____ 57

*SMOOTHIE RECIPES:*_____ *58*

Recipe 1: Berry Blast Smoothie _____ 58

Recipe 2: Green Goodness Smoothie _____ 58

Recipe 3: Tropical Delight Smoothie _____ 58

Recipe 4: Creamy Avocado Smoothie_____ 59

Recipe 5: Almond Butter Banana Smoothie _____ 59

Recipe 6: Mocha Protein Smoothie _____ 60

Recipe 7: Spinach and Pineapple Smoothie _____ 60

Recipe 8: Blueberry Almond Smoothie _____ 61

Recipe 9: Carrot and Ginger Juice _____ 61

Recipe 10: Cucumber and Mint Juice _____ 61

Recipe 11: Beet and Apple Juice_____ 62

Recipe 12: Spinach and Celery Juice _____ 62

Recipe 13: Kale and Pineapple Juice_____ 62

Recipe 14: Apple and Lemon Juice _____ 63

Recipe 15: Tomato and Basil Juice _____ 63

Recipe 16: Spinach and Apple Juice_____ 63

Recipe 17: Ginger and Lemon Infused Water _____ 64

Recipe 18: Cucumber and Lime Infused Water _____ 64

Recipe 19: Watermelon and Mint Infused Water_____ 65

Recipe 20: Strawberry and Basil Infused Water_____ 65

7-day Easy-to-follow Meal Plan for Seniors with Stage 3 Kidney Disease. _____ *66*

EXPERT ADVICE ON MANAGING KIDNEY DISEASE _____ 71

    Medications and Supplements _____ 71

    ACE Inhibitors and ARBs _____ 71

    Diuretics _____ 72

    Erythropoiesis-Stimulating Agents (ESAs) _____ 72

    Phosphate Binders _____ 72

    Vitamin D Supplements _____ 73

    Lifestyle Considerations _____ 73

    Exercise and Lifestyle Changes _____ 73

    How to Monitor Your Kidney Health _____ 74

Tips for Staying Healthy and Active _____ *77*

Foods to Avoid for Kidney Health _____ *82*

INTRODUCTION

Hey there!
If you're holding this book, chances are you or someone you care about is on a journey with kidney disease. I want to start by saying, you're not alone. Navigating the complexities of kidney health can feel like a winding road, but with the right knowledge and support, you can make a real difference in your well-being.

So, what's the deal with kidney disease, anyway? Well, it's a condition that affects millions of people around the world, and it's no small matter. Your kidneys are like the unsung heroes of your body, quietly working behind the scenes to filter waste and regulate crucial elements in your blood. When they're not functioning at their best, it can impact your overall health and vitality.
In this book, we're going to focus on a specific stage: Stage 3 kidney disease. It's a critical juncture, a point where proactive steps in managing your diet can truly make a difference. We'll delve into the nitty-gritty of what that means and how you can embrace a diet that supports your kidney health while still savoring delicious meals.

You might be wondering, why is diet such a big deal when it comes to kidney health? Well, think of it this way: food is like fuel for your body. Just like a car runs best on high-quality gas, your kidneys thrive when you provide them with the right nutrients. But don't worry, this isn't about depriving yourself or embarking on a bland culinary journey. It's about making smart, informed choices that can enhance your well-being.

Throughout these pages, you'll find a treasure trove of kidney-friendly recipes that are not only nutritious but also downright tasty. We're talking breakfasts that kickstart your day, lunches and dinners that satisfy the heartiest of appetites, and snacks and desserts that prove eating well can be a delight.

But it's not just about recipes. We'll also explore meal plans that take the guesswork out of your day, expert advice on managing kidney disease, and tips for staying active and healthy. We're in this together, and I'm here to guide you every step of the way.

So, settle in, grab a cup of something comforting, and let's embark on this journey toward better kidney health. Remember, this book is your companion, filled with knowledge, support, and a whole lot of flavor. Here's to living our best lives with kidney disease!

Warmest regards,
THE KITCHEN SAGE.

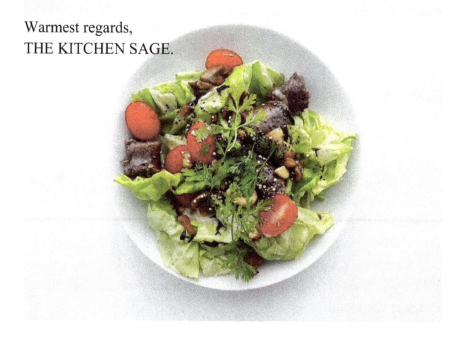

Chapter 1: KIDNEY DISEASE DIET BASICS

Alright, let's dive right in! In this chapter, we'll be unraveling the mysteries of kidney disease, especially at Stage 3. We'll talk about what it is, how your diet plays a starring role, and why eating well is the cornerstone of managing kidney health. Plus, I'll give you a sneak peek of what's coming up in this book.

What is Kidney Disease and Stage 3 Kidney Disease?

Picture your kidneys as diligent little filters in your body's backstage crew. They sift through your blood, removing waste and excess fluids, ensuring everything runs smoothly. But sometimes, due to various reasons like high blood pressure or diabetes, these trusty filters start to sputter. This is when we venture into the territory of kidney disease.

Now, Stage 3 kidney disease? That's where things get interesting. It's like a turning point in the plot. At this stage, your kidneys are working at a reduced capacity, but they're still putting in the effort. Understanding this juncture is crucial because it's precisely here that you can make a tangible difference in your kidney health through smart dietary choices.

How Does Diet Affect Kidney Disease?

Alright, let's get to the heart of the matter ~why does diet matter so much in kidney health? Think of it this way: your kidneys process every morsel that enters your body. They're like the gatekeepers, deciding what stays and what goes. When you're dealing with kidney disease, it's essential to give them a break, or rather, give them the right kind of work.

Certain nutrients can be a bit too much for your kidneys to handle, while others are like high-fives for these vital organs. We're going to talk about which foods fall into which category, so you can make informed decisions about what goes on your plate.

The Importance of Eating Well with Kidney Disease

Alright, let's set the record straight: eating well doesn't mean sacrificing taste or enjoyment. In fact, it's quite the opposite. When you eat in a way that supports your kidney health, you're giving your body the best chance to thrive. It's like providing a tailor-made toolkit for your kidneys to do their job effectively.

We're talking about more energy, better management of blood pressure, and an overall feeling of well-being. So, consider this not just a diet, but a blueprint for feeling your best while managing kidney disease.

What to Expect in This Book

Now, let's talk about what's in store for you. We're not just about theory here ~we're about practical, actionable steps. You can expect a treasure trove of delicious, kidney-friendly recipes that will make your taste buds dance. We'll guide you through meal plans that take the guesswork out of your day. And don't worry, I've got expert advice on managing kidney disease that's going to make your journey a whole lot smoother.

So, grab your apron and let's get started. It's time to embark on a journey of flavor, health, and empowerment in managing your kidney health.

Cheers to vibrant health and delicious meals!

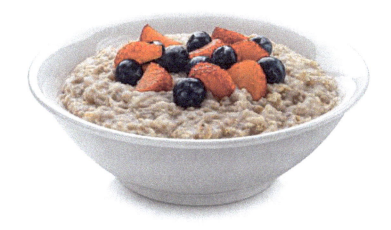

CHAPTER 2: What Nutrients are Important for People with Kidney Disease?

Alright, let's get down to the nitty-gritty of what your kidneys are looking for in their ideal menu. First up, we've got protein. Now, this is a bit of a double-edged sword. On one hand, your body needs it for muscle repair and overall functioning. On the other, too much can put a strain on your kidneys. So, it's all about finding that sweet spot.

Next, let's talk about sodium. Think of it as the sneaky ninja in your diet. Too much, and it can lead to high blood pressure and extra stress on your kidneys. So, we're going to be mindful of where it's hiding.

Then there's phosphorus. Now, this one's a bit of a tricky character. Too much can throw off the delicate balance in your blood, but too little isn't good either. We're going to keep an eye on it and make sure you're getting just the right amount.

And let's not forget about potassium. It's like the conductor of your body's electrical orchestra. But when you've got kidney issues, too much can lead to heart irregularities. So, we'll be balancing it out.

Lastly, we've got fluids. Now, this one's a bit of a dance. Too much and your kidneys might feel overwhelmed. Too little and you're risking dehydration. We're going to find that sweet spot and keep you in perfect harmony.

What Nutrients Should Be Limited?

Alright, let's talk about the rogues' gallery ~the nutrients we need to keep an eye on. First up, it's sodium again. It's like that overzealous friend who just doesn't know when to stop. Too much of it can lead to water retention and high blood pressure. So, we'll be giving it a gentle nudge to step back.

Next, we've got phosphorus. This one tends to hide in some unexpected places, like processed foods and sodas. Too much of it can throw off the balance in your blood, so we'll be keeping tabs on it.

Then there's potassium. Don't get me wrong, it's crucial for nerve and muscle function. But when you've got kidney issues, too much can lead to some unwanted complications. So, we're going to be mindful of where it's showing up.

And let's not forget about protein. Like I said earlier, it's a bit of a balancing act. Too much can put extra stress on your kidneys, so we'll be aiming for just the right amount.

How to Read Food Labels

Now, let's talk about decoding those labels on the back of your favorite foods. It's like learning a secret language that tells you exactly what you're putting into your body.

First up, check out the sodium content. This one's a biggie. Look for foods with lower sodium levels to keep your blood pressure in check.

Next, flip to the phosphorus. It's often listed as an additive, so keep an eye out for names like "phos" or "phosphate". This way, you can keep your phosphorus levels right where they need to be.

Then, take a peek at the potassium. It's not always front and center, so you might have to do a bit of sleuthing. Look for words like "potassium chloride" or "potassium bicarbonate".

And of course, keep an eye on the protein content. It's usually listed right there in plain sight. This way, you can make sure you're giving your kidneys just the right amount of work.

Tips for Cooking Kidney-Friendly Meals

Alright, let's hit the kitchen and whip up some kidney-friendly magic! First off, let's talk about portion sizes. It's all about balance. We're going to be mindful of how much we're putting on our plates to give those kidneys a breather.

Next, let's talk about cooking methods. We're going to be best buddies with methods like baking, grilling, and steaming. They're gentler on your **INGREDIENTS:** and still pack a flavorful punch.

Then there's seasoning. We're going to become best pals with herbs, spices, and citrus. They're going to be your secret weapons for adding flavor without going overboard on sodium.And let's not forget about meal planning. It's like having a roadmap for your week. We're going to plan ahead, make smart choices, and set you up for success in managing your kidney health.

So, get ready to rock that apron and let's create some kidney-friendly culinary masterpieces!

DELICIOUS BREAKFAST RECIPES

Recipe 1: Creamy Oatmeal with Berries

INGREDIENTS:
~1/2 cup rolled oats
~1 cup water
~2 tablespoons low-fat milk
~1/4 cup fresh mixed berries (strawberries, blueberries, raspberries)
~1 tablespoon honey (optional)

PREPARATION METHOD
1. In a saucepan, combine rolled oats and water. Bring to a gentle boil and simmer for 3-5 minutes, stirring occasionally.
2. Once the oats are creamy, stir in the low-fat milk.
3. Transfer the oatmeal to a bowl and top with fresh mixed berries. Drizzle with honey if desired.

Recipe 2: Greek Yogurt Parfait

INGREDIENTS:
~1/2 cup low-fat Greek yogurt
~2 tablespoons chopped nuts (almonds, walnuts)
~1/4 cup fresh mixed berries

~1 tablespoon honey

PREPARATION METHOD
1. In a glass or bowl, layer Greek yogurt, chopped nuts, and fresh mixed berries.
2. Drizzle with honey for added sweetness.

Recipe 3: Scrambled Egg Whites with Spinach and Tomatoes

INGREDIENTS:
~2 egg whites
~1/4 cup chopped spinach
~2 tablespoons diced tomatoes
~Salt and pepper to taste

PREPARATION METHOD
1. In a non-stick pan, lightly sauté chopped spinach and diced tomatoes until softened.
2. Whisk the egg whites and pour them into the pan with the vegetables.
3. Gently scramble until cooked through. Season with salt and pepper.

Recipe 4: Cottage Cheese Pancakes

INGREDIENTS:
~1/2 cup low-fat cottage cheese
~2 tablespoons whole wheat flour
~1 egg

~1/4 teaspoon vanilla extract
~1/4 teaspoon cinnamon
~1/4 cup fresh berries for topping

PREPARATION METHOD

1. In a bowl, combine cottage cheese, whole wheat flour, egg, vanilla extract, and cinnamon. Mix until well combined.
2. Heat a non-stick skillet and spoon batter to form small pancakes. Cook until golden brown on both sides.
3. Top with fresh berries before serving.

Recipe 5: Spinach and Feta Omelette

INGREDIENTS:
~2 eggs
~2 tablespoons chopped spinach
~1 tablespoon crumbled feta cheese
~Salt and pepper to taste

PREPARATION METHOD

1. Whisk eggs in a bowl and pour into a heated non-stick pan.
2. Sprinkle chopped spinach and crumbled feta cheese over one side of the omelette. Fold in half.
3. Cook until the eggs are fully set. Season with salt and pepper.

Recipe 6: Whole Grain Toast with Avocado and Poached Egg

INGREDIENTS:
~1 slice whole grain bread
~1/4 avocado, mashed

~1 poached egg
~Salt and pepper to taste
PREPARATION METHOD
1. Toast the whole grain bread to your desired level of crispiness.
2. Spread mashed avocado evenly on the toast.
3. Place the poached egg on top. Season with salt and pepper.

Recipe 7: Apple Cinnamon Quinoa Bowl

INGREDIENTS:
~1/2 cup cooked quinoa
~1/4 cup unsweetened applesauce
~1/4 teaspoon cinnamon
~1 tablespoon chopped almonds
PREPARATION METHOD
1. In a bowl, combine cooked quinoa, unsweetened applesauce, and cinnamon.
2. Top with chopped almonds for crunch and additional nutrients.

Recipe 8: Sweet Potato and Spinach Hash

INGREDIENTS:
~1/2 cup diced sweet potato
~1/4 cup chopped spinach
~1/4 teaspoon paprika
~1/4 teaspoon garlic powder

~1 teaspoon olive oil

PREPARATION METHOD

1. In a skillet, heat olive oil and add diced sweet potato. Cook until softened and lightly browned.
2. Add chopped spinach, paprika, and garlic powder. Cook until spinach wilts.

Recipe 9: Chia Seed Pudding with Almonds and Berries

INGREDIENTS:

~2 tablespoons chia seeds
~1/2 cup unsweetened almond milk
~1 tablespoon sliced almonds
~1/4 cup fresh mixed berries

PREPARATION METHOD

1. Mix chia seeds and almond milk in a bowl. Let it sit for at least 2 hours or overnight, stirring occasionally.
2. Top with sliced almonds and fresh mixed berries before serving.

Recipe 10: Muesli with Greek Yogurt and Honey

INGREDIENTS:

~1/4 cup muesli
~1/2 cup low-fat Greek yogurt
~1 tablespoon honey

PREPARATION METHOD
1. Combine muesli and Greek yogurt in a bowl.
2. Drizzle with honey for natural sweetness.

Recipe 11: Almond Butter and Banana Wrap

INGREDIENTS:
~1 whole wheat tortilla
~1 tablespoon almond butter
~1/2 banana, sliced

PREPARATION METHOD
1. Spread almond butter on the whole wheat tortilla.
2. Place banana slices in the center and wrap it up.

Recipe 12: Berry Blast Smoothie

INGREDIENTS:
~1/2 cup mixed berries (strawberries, blueberries, raspberries)
~1/2 cup low-fat Greek yogurt
~1/4 cup unsweetened almond milk
~1 tablespoon chia seeds

PREPARATION METHOD
1. Blend mixed berries, Greek yogurt, almond milk, and chia seeds until smooth.

Recipe 13: Spinach and Feta Breakfast Burrito

INGREDIENTS:
~1 whole wheat tortilla
~2 eggs, scrambled
~2 tablespoons chopped spinach
~1 tablespoon crumbled feta cheese

PREPARATION METHOD
1. Lay out the whole wheat tortilla and fill with scrambled eggs, chopped spinach, and crumbled feta cheese.
2. Roll it up into a burrito.

Recipe 14: Banana Nut Overnight Oats

INGREDIENTS:
~1/2 cup rolled oats
~1/2 cup unsweetened almond milk
~1/2 banana, mashed
~1 tablespoon chopped walnuts

PREPARATION METHOD
1. In a jar, combine rolled oats, almond milk, mashed banana, and chopped walnuts. Mix well.
2. Refrigerate overnight and enjoy in the morning.

Recipe 15: Veggie and Cheese Omelette

INGREDIENTS:
~2 eggs
~2 tablespoons chopped bell peppers
~2 tablespoons chopped tomatoes
~2 tablespoons shredded low-fat cheese

PREPARATION METHOD
1. Whisk eggs in a bowl and pour into a heated non-stick pan.
2. Sprinkle bell peppers, tomatoes, and shredded cheese over one side of the omelette. Fold in half.
3. Cook until the eggs are fully set.

Recipe 16: Cinnamon Raisin Toast with Cottage Cheese

INGREDIENTS:
~1 slice whole grain cinnamon raisin bread
~1/4 cup low-fat cottage cheese

PREPARATION METHOD
1. Toast the cinnamon raisin bread to your desired level of crispiness.
2. Spread low-fat cottage cheese evenly on the toast.

Recipe 17: Pineapple and Cottage Cheese Bowl

INGREDIENTS:
~1/2 cup pineapple chunks (fresh or canned in juice)
~1/4 cup low-fat cottage cheese
~1 tablespoon chopped mint leaves
PREPARATION METHOD
1. Combine pineapple chunks and low-fat cottage cheese in a bowl.
2. Garnish with chopped mint leaves for a refreshing touch.

Recipe 18: Avocado and Tomato Toast with Poached Egg

INGREDIENTS:
~1 slice whole grain bread
~1/4 avocado, sliced
~2 slices tomato
~1 poached egg
~Salt and pepper to taste
PREPARATION METHOD
1. Toast the whole grain bread to your desired level of crispiness.
2. Layer sliced avocado and tomato on top.
3. Place the poached egg on top. Season with salt and pepper.

Recipe 19: Blueberry Almond Smoothie Bowl

INGREDIENTS:
~1/2 cup frozen blueberries
~1/2 cup low-fat Greek yogurt
~1 tablespoon almond butter
~1 tablespoon sliced almonds

PREPARATION METHOD
1. Blend frozen blueberries, Greek yogurt, and almond butter until smooth.
2. Pour into a bowl and top with sliced almonds.

Recipe 20: Spinach and Mushroom Frittata

INGREDIENTS:
~4 eggs
~1/4 cup chopped spinach
~1/4 cup sliced mushrooms
~2 tablespoons diced onions
~Salt and pepper to taste

PREPARATION METHOD
1. Preheat oven to 350°F (175°C).
2. In an oven-proof skillet, sauté diced onions until translucent. Add sliced mushrooms and chopped spinach, cooking until wilted.

3. In a bowl, whisk eggs and pour over the vegetables in the skillet. Cook on the stovetop for a few minutes, then transfer to the preheated oven to finish cooking until set.

Enjoy these delicious and kidney-friendly breakfast options! Remember to consult with us through our Email address for personalized dietary advice.

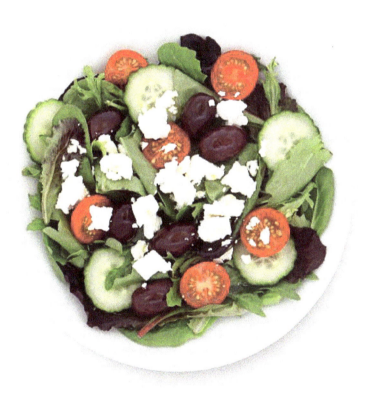

EASY AND DELICIOUS LUNCH RECIPES

Recipe 1: Grilled Salmon Salad

INGREDIENTS:
~4 oz grilled salmon fillet
~2 cups mixed salad greens
~1/4 cup cherry tomatoes, halved
~2 tablespoons cucumber, sliced
~1 tablespoon balsamic vinaigrette

PREPARATION METHOD
1. Place grilled salmon on a bed of mixed salad greens.
2. Add cherry tomatoes and cucumber slices.
3. Drizzle with balsamic vinaigrette.

Recipe 2: Quinoa and Vegetable Stir-Fry

INGREDIENTS:
~1/2 cup cooked quinoa
~1/2 cup mixed vegetables (bell peppers, broccoli, snap peas)
~2 tablespoons low-sodium soy sauce
~1 tablespoon olive oil

PREPARATION METHOD
1. In a heated pan, add olive oil and stir-fry mixed vegetables until tender.
2. Add cooked quinoa and soy sauce, tossing to combine.

Recipe 3: Turkey and Avocado Wrap

INGREDIENTS:
~3 oz cooked turkey breast, sliced
~1/4 avocado, sliced
~1 whole wheat tortilla
~1 tablespoon hummus

PREPARATION METHOD
1. Spread hummus on the whole wheat tortilla.
2. Layer sliced turkey and avocado, then wrap it up.

Recipe 4: Spinach and Chickpea Salad

INGREDIENTS:
~1 cup baby spinach leaves
~1/2 cup canned chickpeas, rinsed and drained
~2 tablespoons feta cheese, crumbled
~1 tablespoon lemon-tahini dressing

PREPARATION METHOD
1. Toss baby spinach with chickpeas and crumbled feta cheese.
2. Drizzle with lemon-tahini dressing.

Recipe 5: Egg Salad Lettuce Wraps

INGREDIENTS:
~2 hard-boiled eggs, chopped
~2 tablespoons Greek yogurt
~1 tablespoon chopped chives
~Lettuce leaves for wrapping

PREPARATION METHOD
1. In a bowl, combine chopped hard-boiled eggs, Greek yogurt, and chives.
2. Spoon the mixture into lettuce leaves for a low-carb wrap.

Recipe 6: Lentil and Vegetable Soup

INGREDIENTS:
~1/2 cup cooked lentils
~1/2 cup mixed vegetables (carrots, celery, zucchini)
~2 cups low-sodium vegetable broth
~1/2 teaspoon dried thyme

PREPARATION METHOD
1. In a pot, combine cooked lentils, mixed vegetables, vegetable broth, and dried thyme. Simmer until vegetables are tender.

Recipe 7: Tuna and White Bean Salad

INGREDIENTS:
~3 oz canned tuna, drained

~1/4 cup canned white beans, rinsed and drained
~2 cups mixed salad greens
~1 tablespoon lemon-tahini dressing
PREPARATION METHOD
1. Combine canned tuna and white beans with mixed salad greens.
2. Drizzle with lemon-tahini dressing.

Recipe 8: Caprese Salad with Balsamic Glaze

INGREDIENTS:
~1 medium tomato, sliced
~2 oz fresh mozzarella, sliced
~Fresh basil leaves
~1 tablespoon balsamic glaze
PREPARATION METHOD
1. Arrange tomato and mozzarella slices on a plate, alternating with basil leaves.
2. Drizzle with balsamic glaze.

Recipe 9: Chicken and Vegetable Skewers

INGREDIENTS:
~3 oz grilled chicken breast, cubed
~1/2 cup bell peppers, diced
~1/2 cup zucchini, sliced
~1 tablespoon olive oil

PREPARATION METHOD
1. Thread grilled chicken, bell peppers, and zucchini onto skewers.
2. Brush with olive oil and grill until cooked through.

Recipe 10: Greek Yogurt Chicken Salad

INGREDIENTS:
~3 oz cooked chicken breast, shredded
~2 tablespoons low-fat Greek yogurt
~1 tablespoon chopped celery
~1 tablespoon chopped walnuts

PREPARATION METHOD
1. In a bowl, mix shredded chicken, Greek yogurt, chopped celery, and chopped walnuts.

Recipe 11: Sweet Potato and Black Bean Bowl

INGREDIENTS:
~1/2 cup roasted sweet potato cubes
~1/4 cup canned black beans, rinsed and drained
~2 tablespoons diced red onion
~1 tablespoon lime-tahini dressing

PREPARATION METHOD
1. Combine roasted sweet potato cubes, black beans, and diced red onion.

2. Drizzle with lime-tahini dressing.

Recipe 12: Spinach and Goat Cheese Stuffed Chicken Breast

INGREDIENTS:
~3 oz chicken breast
~1/4 cup fresh spinach leaves
~1 tablespoon goat cheese
~Salt and pepper to taste
PREPARATION METHOD
1. Preheat oven to 375°F (190°C).
2. Cut a pocket into the side of the chicken breast and stuff with fresh spinach leaves and goat cheese. Season with salt and pepper.
3. Bake until chicken is cooked through.

Recipe 13: Cauliflower and Broccoli Soup

INGREDIENTS:
~1/2 cup cauliflower florets
~1/2 cup broccoli florets
~2 cups low-sodium vegetable broth
~1/4 teaspoon turmeric
PREPARATION METHOD
1. In a pot, combine cauliflower and broccoli florets with vegetable broth and turmeric. Simmer until vegetables are tender.
2. Blend until smooth.

Recipe 14: Shrimp and Asparagus Stir-Fry

INGREDIENTS:
~3 oz cooked shrimp
~1/2 cup asparagus spears, sliced
~2 tablespoons low-sodium soy sauce
~1 tablespoon olive oil

PREPARATION METHOD
1. In a heated pan, add olive oil and stir-fry asparagus until tender.
2. Add cooked shrimp and soy sauce, tossing to combine.

Recipe 15: Chickpea and Avocado Salad

INGREDIENTS:
~1/2 cup canned chickpeas, rinsed and drained
~1/4 avocado, diced
~2 tablespoons diced cucumber
~1 tablespoon lemon-tahini dressing

PREPARATION METHOD
1. Combine chickpeas, diced avocado, and diced cucumber in a bowl.
2. Drizzle with lemon-tahini dressing.

Recipe 16: Broccoli and Cheddar Stuffed Sweet Potato

INGREDIENTS:
~1 small sweet potato, baked
~1/2 cup steamed broccoli florets
~2 tablespoons shredded cheddar cheese

PREPARATION METHOD
1. Slice open the baked sweet potato and fluff the insides with a fork.
2. Stuff with steamed broccoli florets and top with shredded cheddar cheese.

Recipe 17: Turkey and Spinach Wrap with Hummus

INGREDIENTS:
~3 oz cooked turkey breast, sliced
~1/2 cup fresh spinach leaves
~1 whole wheat tortilla
~1 tablespoon hummus

PREPARATION METHOD
1. Spread hummus on the whole wheat tortilla.
2. Layer sliced turkey and fresh spinach, then wrap it up.

Recipe 18: Tomato Basil Mozzarella Salad

INGREDIENTS:
~1 medium tomato, sliced
~2 oz fresh mozzarella, sliced
~Fresh basil leaves
~1 tablespoon olive oil

PREPARATION METHOD
1. Arrange tomato and mozzarella slices on a plate, alternating with basil leaves.
2. Drizzle with olive oil.

Recipe 19: Tofu and Vegetable Stir-Fry

INGREDIENTS:
~1/2 cup cubed firm tofu
~1/2 cup mixed vegetables (broccoli, carrots, snap peas)
~2 tablespoons low-sodium soy sauce
~1 tablespoon sesame oil

PREPARATION METHOD
1. In a heated pan, add sesame oil and stir-fry tofu and mixed vegetables until heated through.
2. Add low-sodium soy sauce and toss to combine.

Recipe 20: Spinach and Feta Stuffed Chicken Breast

INGREDIENTS:
~3 oz chicken breast
~1/4 cup chopped spinach
~1 tablespoon crumbled feta cheese
~Salt and pepper to taste

PREPARATION METHOD
1. Preheat oven to 375°F (190°C).
2. Cut a pocket into the side of the chicken breast and stuff with chopped spinach and crumbled feta cheese. Season with salt and pepper.
3. Bake until chicken is cooked through.

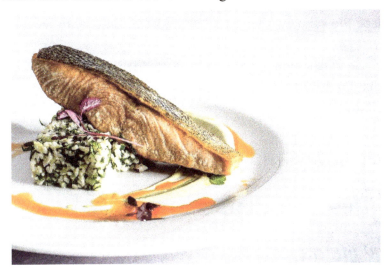

QUICK AND EASY DINNER RECIPES

Recipe 1: Baked Lemon Herb Salmon

INGREDIENTS:
~4 oz salmon fillet
~1 tablespoon lemon juice
~1/2 teaspoon dried dill
~Salt and pepper to taste
PREPARATION METHOD
1. Preheat the oven to 375°F (190°C).
2. Place the salmon fillet on a baking sheet lined with parchment paper.
3. Drizzle with lemon juice, sprinkle with dried dill, salt, and pepper.
4. Bake for 15-20 minutes or until the salmon flakes easily with a fork.

Recipe 2: Spinach and Tomato Stuffed Bell Peppers

INGREDIENTS:
~2 medium bell peppers, halved and seeded
~1/2 cup cooked quinoa
~1/4 cup chopped spinach

~1/4 cup diced tomatoes
~2 tablespoons shredded mozzarella cheese

PREPARATION METHOD

1. Preheat the oven to 350°F (175°C).
2. In a bowl, mix cooked quinoa, chopped spinach, diced tomatoes, and mozzarella cheese.
3. Stuff the bell pepper halves with the mixture and place in a baking dish.
4. Bake for 25-30 minutes or until peppers are tender.

Recipe 3: Turkey and Vegetable Stir-Fry

INGREDIENTS:

~3 oz cooked turkey breast, sliced
~1/2 cup mixed vegetables (bell peppers, broccoli, carrots)
~2 tablespoons low-sodium soy sauce
~1 tablespoon olive oil

PREPARATION METHOD

1. In a heated pan, add olive oil and stir-fry mixed vegetables until tender.
2. Add sliced turkey and low-sodium soy sauce, tossing to combine.

Recipe 4: Cauliflower Rice with Shrimp and Peas

INGREDIENTS:

~1/2 cup cauliflower rice

~3 oz cooked shrimp
~1/4 cup peas
~1 tablespoon chopped parsley

PREPARATION METHOD

1. Steam cauliflower rice until tender.
2. In a separate pan, sauté cooked shrimp and peas until heated through.
3. Combine cauliflower rice with shrimp and peas. Top with chopped parsley.

Recipe 5: Eggplant and Tomato Caprese

INGREDIENTS:

~1 medium eggplant, sliced
~1 medium tomato, sliced
~2 oz fresh mozzarella, sliced
~Fresh basil leaves
~1 tablespoon balsamic glaze

PREPARATION METHOD

1. Preheat the grill or grill pan.
2. Grill eggplant slices until tender, about 3-4 minutes per side.
3. Layer grilled eggplant, tomato, mozzarella, and basil leaves on a plate. Drizzle with balsamic glaze.

Recipe 6: Chicken and Vegetable Skillet

INGREDIENTS:
~3 oz cooked chicken breast, cubed
~1/2 cup mixed vegetables (zucchini, bell peppers, carrots)
~1 tablespoon olive oil
~1/2 teaspoon dried Italian herbs

PREPARATION METHOD
1. In a skillet, heat olive oil and add mixed vegetables. Sauté until tender.
2. Add cubed chicken and dried Italian herbs, tossing to combine.

Recipe 7: Stuffed Portobello Mushrooms

INGREDIENTS:
~2 large portobello mushrooms, stems removed
~1/4 cup cooked quinoa
~1/4 cup chopped spinach
~2 tablespoons shredded mozzarella cheese

PREPARATION METHOD
1. Preheat the oven to 375°F (190°C).
2. In a bowl, mix cooked quinoa, chopped spinach, and mozzarella cheese.
3. Stuff the portobello mushrooms with the mixture and place on a baking sheet.
4. Bake for 20-25 minutes or until mushrooms are tender.

Recipe 8: Beef and Broccoli Stir-Fry

INGREDIENTS:
~3 oz lean beef, thinly sliced
~1/2 cup broccoli florets
~2 tablespoons low-sodium soy sauce
~1 tablespoon sesame oil

PREPARATION METHOD
1. In a heated pan, add sesame oil and stir-fry beef until browned.
2. Add broccoli florets and low-sodium soy sauce, tossing to combine.

Recipe 9: Zucchini Noodles with Pesto and Cherry Tomatoes

INGREDIENTS:
~1 medium zucchini, spiralized into noodles
~2 tablespoons pesto sauce
~1/4 cup cherry tomatoes, halved
~1 tablespoon grated Parmesan cheese

PREPARATION METHOD
1. In a pan, sauté zucchini noodles with pesto sauce until heated through.
2. Add cherry tomatoes and cook for an additional 2 minutes.
3. Top with grated Parmesan cheese before serving.

Recipe 10: Greek Chicken and Vegetable Skewers

INGREDIENTS:
~3 oz grilled chicken breast, cubed
~1/2 cup mixed vegetables (zucchini, bell peppers, red onion)
~1 tablespoon olive oil
~1/2 teaspoon dried oregano

PREPARATION METHOD
1. Thread grilled chicken and mixed vegetables onto skewers.
2. Brush with olive oil and sprinkle with dried oregano.
3. Grill until chicken is cooked through.

Recipe 11: Lentil and Spinach Curry

INGREDIENTS:
~1/2 cup cooked lentils
~1/2 cup chopped spinach
~1/4 cup diced tomatoes
~2 tablespoons coconut milk
~1/2 teaspoon curry powder

PREPARATION METHOD
1. In a pot, combine cooked lentils, chopped spinach, diced tomatoes, coconut milk, and curry powder. Simmer until heated through.

Recipe 12: Baked Chicken Thighs with Herbs

INGREDIENTS:
~2 bone-in chicken thighs
~1/2 teaspoon dried rosemary
~1/2 teaspoon dried thyme
~Salt and pepper to taste
PREPARATION METHOD
1. Preheat the oven to 375°F (190°C).
2. Season chicken thighs with dried rosemary, dried thyme, salt, and pepper.
3. Place on a baking sheet and bake for 30-35 minutes or until cooked through.

Recipe 13: Tomato and Spinach Frittata

INGREDIENTS:
~4 eggs
~1/4 cup diced tomatoes
~1/4 cup chopped spinach
~2 tablespoons grated Parmesan cheese
PREPARATION METHOD
1. Preheat the oven to 350°F (175°C).
2. Whisk eggs in a bowl and stir in diced tomatoes, chopped spinach, and grated Parmesan cheese.

3. Pour mixture into a greased oven-proof skillet and bake for 15-20 minutes or until set.

Recipe 14: Tofu and Vegetable Curry

INGREDIENTS:
~1/2 cup cubed firm tofu
~1/2 cup mixed vegetables (eggplant, bell peppers, snap peas)
~2 tablespoons coconut milk
~1/2 teaspoon curry powder

PREPARATION METHOD
1. In a pot, combine cubed tofu, mixed vegetables, coconut milk, and curry powder. Simmer until heated through.

Recipe 15: Spaghetti Squash with Tomato Sauce

INGREDIENTS:
~1 cup cooked spaghetti squash
~1/4 cup tomato sauce (low-sodium)
~2 tablespoons grated Parmesan cheese
~Fresh basil leaves for garnish

PREPARATION METHOD
1. Heat cooked spaghetti squash in a pan with tomato sauce until heated through.
2. Top with grated Parmesan cheese and fresh basil leaves.

Recipe 16: Shrimp and Asparagus Bake

INGREDIENTS:
~3 oz cooked shrimp
~1/2 cup asparagus spears, trimmed
~1 tablespoon olive oil
~1/2 teaspoon dried Italian herbs
PREPARATION METHOD
1. Preheat the oven to 375°F (190°C).
2. Toss cooked shrimp and asparagus with olive oil and dried Italian herbs.
3. Place on a baking sheet and bake for 10-12 minutes or until shrimp are heated through.

Recipe 17: Spinach and Feta Stuffed Turkey Burger

INGREDIENTS:
~3 oz lean ground turkey
~1/4 cup chopped spinach
~1 tablespoon crumbled feta cheese
~Salt and pepper to taste
PREPARATION METHOD
1. Mix lean ground turkey, chopped spinach, crumbled feta cheese, salt, and pepper in a bowl.
2. Form into a patty and grill until cooked through.

Recipe 18: Broccoli and Cheddar Stuffed Chicken Thigh

INGREDIENTS:
~2 bone-in chicken thighs
~1/2 cup steamed broccoli florets
~2 tablespoons shredded cheddar cheese

PREPARATION METHOD
1. Preheat the oven to 375°F (190°C).
2. Cut a pocket into the side of the chicken thighs and stuff with steamed broccoli florets and shredded cheddar cheese.
3. Bake for 30-35 minutes or until chicken is cooked through.

Recipe 19: Caprese Stuffed Portobello Mushrooms

INGREDIENTS:
~2 large portobello mushrooms, stems removed
~1 medium tomato, sliced
~2 oz fresh mozzarella, sliced
~Fresh basil leaves
~1 tablespoon balsamic glaze

PREPARATION METHOD
1. Preheat the oven to 375°F (190°C).
2. Grill portobello mushrooms for 3-4 minutes per side.
3. Layer grilled mushrooms with tomato, mozzarella, and basil leaves. Drizzle with balsamic glaze.

Recipe 20: Pesto Zucchini Noodles with Grilled Chicken

INGREDIENTS:
~1 medium zucchini, spiralized into noodles
~3 oz grilled chicken breast, sliced
~2 tablespoons pesto sauce
~1 tablespoon grated Parmesan cheese

PREPARATION METHOD
1. In a pan, sauté zucchini noodles with pesto sauce until heated through.
2. Add sliced grilled chicken and cook for an additional 2 minutes.
3. Top with grated Parmesan cheese before serving.

Enjoy these delicious and kidney-friendly dinner options!

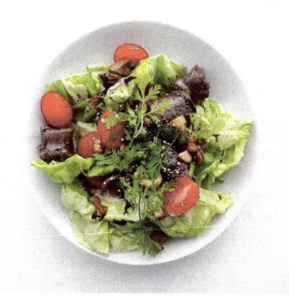

DELICIOUS SNACKS AND DESSERT RECIPES

Snacks:

Recipe 1: Cucumber and Hummus Bites

INGREDIENTS:
~1 small cucumber, sliced
~2 tablespoons hummus
PREPARATION METHOD
1. Spread a small amount of hummus on each cucumber slice.
2. Serve as bite-sized snacks.

Recipe 2: Greek Yogurt with Berries

INGREDIENTS:
~1/2 cup low-fat Greek yogurt
~1/4 cup fresh mixed berries
PREPARATION METHOD
1. Top Greek yogurt with fresh mixed berries.

Recipe 3: Almonds and Dried Apricots

INGREDIENTS:
~1/4 cup almonds
~2 dried apricots
PREPARATION METHOD
1. Combine almonds and dried apricots for a satisfying and nutritious snack.

Recipe 4: Cottage Cheese with Pineapple

INGREDIENTS:
~1/4 cup low-fat cottage cheese
~1/4 cup pineapple chunks (fresh or canned in juice)
PREPARATION METHOD:
1. Combine cottage cheese with pineapple chunks.

Recipe 5: Baked Sweet Potato Fries

INGREDIENTS:
~1 small sweet potato, cut into fries
~1 teaspoon olive oil
~1/4 teaspoon garlic powder
PREPARATION METHOD:
1. Preheat the oven to 425°F (220°C).

2. Toss sweet potato fries with olive oil and garlic powder. Spread on a baking sheet.
3. Bake for 20-25 minutes or until crispy.

Recipe 6: Hard-Boiled Eggs with Paprika

INGREDIENTS:
~2 hard-boiled eggs
~Pinch of paprika
PREPARATION METHOD:
1. Slice hard-boiled eggs in half and sprinkle with a pinch of paprika.

Recipe 7: Rice Cake with Almond Butter and Banana

INGREDIENTS:
~1 rice cake
~1 tablespoon almond butter
~1/2 banana, sliced
PREPARATION METHOD:
1. Spread almond butter on the rice cake and top with banana slices.

Recipe 8: Carrot Sticks with Hummus

INGREDIENTS:
~1 medium carrot, cut into sticks
~2 tablespoons hummus
PREPARATION METHOD:
1. Dip carrot sticks into hummus for a crunchy and nutritious snack.

Recipe 9: Berry Parfait

INGREDIENTS:
~1/2 cup low-fat Greek yogurt
~1/4 cup fresh mixed berries
~1 tablespoon honey (optional)
PREPARATION METHOD:
1. In a glass, layer Greek yogurt and fresh mixed berries. Drizzle with honey if desired.

Recipe 10: Baked Apple with Cinnamon

INGREDIENTS:
~1 small apple
~1/2 teaspoon cinnamon
PREPARATION METHOD:
1. Core the apple and sprinkle with cinnamon. Place in a baking dish.

2. Bake at 350°F (175°C) for 20-25 minutes or until tender.

Recipe 11: Chia Seed Pudding with Almonds and Berries

INGREDIENTS:
~2 tablespoons chia seeds
~1/2 cup unsweetened almond milk
~1 tablespoon sliced almonds
~1/4 cup fresh mixed berries

PREPARATION METHOD:
1. Mix chia seeds and almond milk in a bowl. Let it sit for at least 2 hours or overnight, stirring occasionally.
2. Top with sliced almonds and fresh mixed berries.

Recipe 12: Banana and Walnut Muffins

INGREDIENTS:
~1/2 ripe banana, mashed
~1/4 cup chopped walnuts
~1/2 cup whole wheat flour
~1/2 teaspoon baking powder
~1 tablespoon honey

PREPARATION METHOD:
1. In a bowl, combine mashed banana, chopped walnuts, whole wheat flour, baking powder, and honey. Mix until well combined.

2. Spoon the mixture into a muffin tin and bake at 350°F (175°C) for 15-20 minutes.

Recipe 13: Dark Chocolate Covered Strawberries

INGREDIENTS:
~4 fresh strawberries
~1 ounce dark chocolate (70% cocoa or higher)
PREPARATION METHOD:
1. Melt dark chocolate in the microwave or on the stovetop using a double boiler.
2. Dip each strawberry into the melted chocolate and place on parchment paper to cool.

Recipe 14: Vanilla Yogurt with Sliced Almonds

INGREDIENTS:
~1/2 cup low-fat vanilla yogurt
~1 tablespoon sliced almonds
PREPARATION METHOD:
1. Top vanilla yogurt with sliced almonds for a simple and satisfying dessert.

Recipe 15: Peach and Cottage Cheese Bowl

INGREDIENTS:
~1/2 cup sliced peaches (fresh or canned in juice)
~1/4 cup low-fat cottage cheese
~1 tablespoon chopped mint leaves

PREPARATION METHOD:
1. Combine sliced peaches and low-fat cottage cheese in a bowl.
2. Garnish with chopped mint leaves for a refreshing touch.

Recipe 16: Oatmeal Raisin Cookies

INGREDIENTS:
~1/2 cup rolled oats
~1/4 cup whole wheat flour
~1/4 cup raisins
~2 tablespoons honey
~1 tablespoon unsweetened applesauce

PREPARATION METHOD:
1. In a bowl, combine rolled oats, whole wheat flour, raisins, honey, and unsweetened applesauce. Mix until well combined.
2. Drop spoonfuls of the mixture onto a baking sheet and bake at 350°F (175°C) for 10-12 minutes.

Recipe 17: Baked Pears with Cinnamon

INGREDIENTS:
~1 medium pear, halved and cored
~1/2 teaspoon cinnamon
~1 tablespoon chopped walnuts
PREPARATION METHOD:
1. Place pear halves in a baking dish, cut side up.
2. Sprinkle with cinnamon and top with chopped walnuts.
3. Bake at 350°F (175°C) for 20-25 minutes or until tender.

Recipe 18: Blueberry Yogurt Parfait

INGREDIENTS:
~1/2 cup low-fat plain yogurt
~1/4 cup fresh blueberries
~1 tablespoon sliced almonds
PREPARATION METHOD:
1. In a glass, layer plain yogurt, fresh blueberries, and sliced almonds.

Recipe 19: Chocolate Banana Smoothie

INGREDIENTS:
~1/2 banana

~1 cup unsweetened almond milk
~1 tablespoon unsweetened cocoa powder
~1 tablespoon honey (optional)
PREPARATION METHOD:
1. Blend banana, almond milk, cocoa powder, and honey (if using) until smooth.

Recipe 20: Apple and Cinnamon Rice Cake

INGREDIENTS:
~1 rice cake
~1/2 small apple, thinly sliced
~Pinch of cinnamon
PREPARATION METHOD:
1. Place apple slices on the rice cake and sprinkle with cinnamon for a sweet treat.

Enjoy these delightful and kidney-friendly snack and dessert options! Remember to consult with our healthcare professionals through our email for personalized dietary advice

SMOOTHIE RECIPES:

Recipe 1: Berry Blast Smoothie

INGREDIENTS:
~1/2 cup mixed berries (blueberries, raspberries, and strawberries)
~1/2 cup low-fat plain yogurt
~1/4 cup unsweetened almond milk
~1 tablespoon honey (optional)
PREPARATION METHOD:
1. Blend mixed berries, plain yogurt, almond milk, and honey (if using) until smooth.

Recipe 2: Green Goodness Smoothie

INGREDIENTS:
~1/2 cup fresh spinach leaves
~1/2 banana
~1/4 cup low-fat plain yogurt
~1/4 cup unsweetened almond milk
PREPARATION METHOD:
1. Blend spinach leaves, banana, plain yogurt, and almond milk until smooth.

Recipe 3: Tropical Delight Smoothie

INGREDIENTS:
~1/2 cup pineapple chunks (fresh or canned in juice)

~1/4 cup low-fat plain yogurt
~1/4 cup unsweetened coconut milk
PREPARATION METHOD:
1. Blend pineapple chunks, plain yogurt, and coconut milk until smooth.

Recipe 4: Creamy Avocado Smoothie

INGREDIENTS:
~1/4 avocado, peeled and pitted
~1/2 cup low-fat plain yogurt
~1/4 cup unsweetened almond milk
~1 tablespoon honey (optional)
PREPARATION METHOD:
1. Blend avocado, plain yogurt, almond milk, and honey (if using) until creamy.

Recipe 5: Almond Butter Banana Smoothie

INGREDIENTS:
~1/2 banana
~1 tablespoon almond butter
~1/2 cup low-fat plain yogurt
~1/4 cup unsweetened almond milk
PREPARATION METHOD:
1. Blend banana, almond butter, plain yogurt, and almond milk until well combined.

Recipe 6: Mocha Protein Smoothie

INGREDIENTS:
~1/2 cup brewed coffee, cooled
~1/4 cup low-fat plain yogurt
~1/4 cup unsweetened almond milk
~1 tablespoon unsweetened cocoa powder
PREPARATION METHOD:
1. Blend brewed coffee, plain yogurt, almond milk, and cocoa powder until smooth.

Recipe 7: Spinach and Pineapple Smoothie

INGREDIENTS:
~1/2 cup fresh spinach leaves
~1/2 cup pineapple chunks (fresh or canned in juice)
~1/4 cup low-fat plain yogurt
~1/4 cup unsweetened almond milk
PREPARATION METHOD:
1. Blend spinach leaves, pineapple chunks, plain yogurt, and almond milk until smooth.

Recipe 8: Blueberry Almond Smoothie

INGREDIENTS:
~1/2 cup frozen blueberries
~1/2 cup low-fat plain yogurt
~1 tablespoon almond butter
~1 tablespoon sliced almonds
PREPARATION METHOD:
1. Blend frozen blueberries, plain yogurt, almond butter, and sliced almonds until smooth.

Recipe 9: Carrot and Ginger Juice

INGREDIENTS:
~2 large carrots
~1-inch piece of fresh ginger
PREPARATION METHOD:
1. Wash and peel the carrots. Trim the ends.
2. Peel the ginger.
3. Run both the carrots and ginger through a juicer.

Recipe 10: Cucumber and Mint Juice

INGREDIENTS:
~1 medium cucumber
~Handful of fresh mint leaves

PREPARATION METHOD:
1. Wash and cut the cucumber into chunks.
2. Wash the mint leaves.
3. Run both the cucumber and mint through a juicer.

Recipe 11: Beet and Apple Juice

INGREDIENTS:
~1 small beet
~1 medium apple
PREPARATION METHOD:
1. Wash and peel the beet. Cut into chunks.
2. Wash and core the apple. Cut into chunks.
3. Run both the beet and apple through a juicer.

Recipe 12: Spinach and Celery Juice

INGREDIENTS:
~Handful of fresh spinach leaves
~2 stalks of celery
PREPARATION METHOD:
1. Wash the spinach leaves and celery stalks.
2. Run both the spinach and celery through a juicer.

Recipe 13: Kale and Pineapple Juice

INGREDIENTS:
~Handful of fresh kale leaves
~1/2 cup pineapple chunks (fresh or canned in juice)

PREPARATION METHOD:
1. Wash the kale leaves.
2. Run both the kale and pineapple chunks through a juicer.

Recipe 14: Apple and Lemon Juice

INGREDIENTS:
~2 medium apples
~Juice of 1/2 lemon
PREPARATION METHOD:
1. Wash and core the apples. Cut into chunks.
2. Squeeze the juice from half a lemon.
3. Run the apples and lemon juice through a juicer.

Recipe 15: Tomato and Basil Juice

INGREDIENTS:
~2 large tomatoes
~Handful of fresh basil leaves
PREPARATION METHOD:
1. Wash the tomatoes and cut into chunks.
2. Wash the basil leaves.
3. Run both the tomatoes and basil through a juicer.

Recipe 16: Spinach and Apple Juice

INGREDIENTS:
~Handful of fresh spinach leaves

-2 medium apples
PREPARATION METHOD:
1. Wash the spinach leaves.
2. Wash and core the apples. Cut into chunks.
3. Run both the spinach and apples through a juicer.

Recipe 17: Ginger and Lemon Infused Water

INGREDIENTS:
~1-inch piece of fresh ginger
~Juice of 1 lemon
~4 cups of water
PREPARATION METHOD:
1. Peel and slice the ginger.
2. Combine ginger slices, lemon juice, and water in a pitcher. Let it infuse for at least 30 minutes before serving.

Recipe 18: Cucumber and Lime Infused Water

INGREDIENTS:
~1 medium cucumber, sliced
~2 limes, sliced
~4 cups of water
PREPARATION METHOD:
1. Combine cucumber slices, lime slices, and water in a pitcher. Let it infuse for at least 30 minutes before serving.

Recipe 19: Watermelon and Mint Infused Water

INGREDIENTS:
~2 cups watermelon chunks
~Handful of fresh mint leaves
~4 cups of water
PREPARATION METHOD:
1. Combine watermelon chunks, mint leaves, and water in a pitcher. Let it infuse for at least 30 minutes before serving.

Recipe 20: Strawberry and Basil Infused Water

INGREDIENTS:
~1 cup fresh strawberries, halved
~Handful of fresh basil leaves
~4 cups of water
PREPARATION METHOD:
1. Combine strawberry halves, basil leaves, and water in a pitcher. Let it infuse for at least 30 minutes before serving.

Enjoy these refreshing and kidney-friendly smoothie and juicing options!

7-day Easy-to-follow Meal Plan for Seniors with Stage 3 Kidney Disease.

Day 1:
Breakfast:
~Berry Blast Smoothie (Recipe 1)
~1 small whole wheat toast with a teaspoon of almond butter

Lunch:
~Spinach and Tomato Stuffed Bell Peppers (Recipe 2)
~Mixed green salad with balsamic vinaigrette

Snack:
~Greek Yogurt with Berries (Recipe 9)

Dinner:
~Baked Lemon Herb Salmon (Recipe 1)
~Steamed asparagus spears
~Quinoa pilaf

Day 2:

Breakfast:
~Green Goodness Smoothie (Recipe 2)

~1 small banana

Lunch:
~Lentil and Spinach Curry (Recipe 11)
~Brown rice

Snack:
~Almonds and Dried Apricots (Recipe 3)

Dinner:
~Beef and Broccoli Stir-Fry (Recipe 8)
~Steamed brown rice

Day 3:

Breakfast:
~Tropical Delight Smoothie (Recipe 3)
~1/4 cup mixed nuts

Lunch:
~Tomato and Spinach Frittata (Recipe 13)
~Mixed green salad with olive oil dressing

Snack:
~Cottage Cheese with Pineapple (Recipe 4)

Dinner:
~Spinach and Feta Stuffed Turkey Burger (Recipe 17)
~Baked sweet potato fries

Day 4:

Breakfast:
~Creamy Avocado Smoothie (Recipe 4)
~1 small whole wheat toast with a teaspoon of jam

Lunch:
~Tofu and Vegetable Stir-Fry (Recipe 19)
~Brown rice

Snack:
~Carrot Sticks with Hummus (Recipe 8)

Dinner:
~Baked Chicken Thighs with Herbs (Recipe 12)
~Steamed broccoli florets
~Quinoa pilaf

Day 5:

Breakfast:
~Almond Butter Banana Smoothie (Recipe 5)
~1 small apple

Lunch:
~Spaghetti Squash with Tomato Sauce (Recipe 15)
~Mixed green salad with balsamic vinaigrette

Snack:
~Hard-Boiled Eggs with Paprika (Recipe 6)

Dinner:
~Caprese Stuffed Portobello Mushrooms (Recipe 19)
~Steamed green beans

Day 6:

Breakfast:
~Mocha Protein Smoothie (Recipe 6)
~1 small banana

Lunch:
~Chicken and Vegetable Skillet (Recipe 6)
~Mixed green salad with olive oil dressing

Snack:
~Rice Cake with Almond Butter and Banana (Recipe 7)

Dinner:
~Spinach and Tomato Stuffed Bell Peppers (Recipe 2)
~Steamed asparagus spears
~Brown rice

Day 7:

Breakfast:
~Blueberry Almond Smoothie (Recipe 8)

~1/4 cup mixed nuts

Lunch:
~Beef and Broccoli Stir-Fry (Recipe 8)
~Brown rice

Snack:
~Almonds and Dried Apricots (Recipe 3)

Dinner:
~Baked Lemon Herb Salmon (Recipe 1)
~Steamed broccoli florets
~Quinoa pilaf

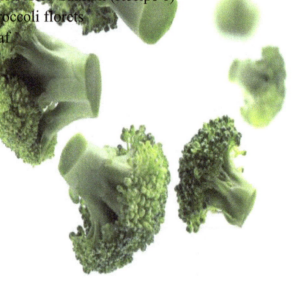

EXPERT ADVICE ON MANAGING KIDNEY DISEASE

Medications and Supplements

Managing kidney disease requires a multi-faceted approach, and medications play a crucial role in maintaining kidney function and overall health. It is imperative to work closely with your healthcare team to determine the right combination of medications tailored to your specific condition. Here, we will explore common medications and supplements used in the management of kidney disease.

ACE Inhibitors and ARBs

Angiotensin-Converting Enzyme (ACE) inhibitors and Angiotensin Receptor Blockers (ARBs) are two classes of medications that are commonly prescribed for individuals with kidney disease. They work by relaxing blood vessels, which helps lower blood pressure and reduce stress on the kidneys. These medications also have the added benefit of reducing proteinuria, a common complication of kidney disease.

Diuretics

Diuretics, also known as water pills, help the kidneys remove excess sodium and water from the body. This can be particularly beneficial for individuals with kidney disease, as it helps regulate blood pressure and fluid balance. However, it is essential to monitor potassium levels, as diuretics can lead to potassium depletion.

Erythropoiesis-Stimulating Agents (ESAs)

For individuals with anemia associated with kidney disease, ESAs may be prescribed. These medications stimulate the production of red blood cells, helping to alleviate fatigue and weakness. Close monitoring of hemoglobin levels is crucial to ensure the medication is effective without causing excessive red blood cell production.

Phosphate Binders

In cases where there is an excess of phosphorus in the blood, phosphate binders may be recommended. These medications work by binding to dietary phosphorus, preventing its absorption in the digestive tract. By controlling phosphorus levels, the risk of complications such as bone disease and calcification of blood vessels is reduced.

Vitamin D Supplements

Kidney disease can lead to reduced activation of vitamin D, which is essential for bone health. Therefore, individuals with kidney disease may be prescribed vitamin D supplements to maintain optimal levels. It is crucial to monitor both calcium and phosphorus levels when taking vitamin D supplements to prevent imbalances.

Lifestyle Considerations

Alongside medications, making positive lifestyle changes is instrumental in managing kidney disease effectively.

Exercise and Lifestyle Changes

Regular Physical Activity

Engaging in regular exercise has numerous benefits for individuals with kidney disease. It helps maintain a healthy weight, regulate blood pressure, and improve overall cardiovascular health. Activities like walking, swimming, and gentle yoga are excellent choices. It is essential to consult with a healthcare professional before starting any exercise program to ensure it is safe and tailored to your specific needs.

Balanced Diet

A kidney-friendly diet is essential in managing kidney disease. This typically involves controlling sodium, potassium, phosphorus, and protein intake. Foods that are rich in antioxidants, such as fruits and vegetables, should be prioritized. It's crucial to work with a registered dietitian who specializes in kidney health to create a personalized meal plan that meets your nutritional needs.

Hydration

Proper hydration is vital for kidney function. It helps flush toxins from the body and maintains optimal blood volume. However, individuals with kidney disease may need to monitor their fluid intake more closely, as excessive fluid retention can be detrimental. Consulting with a healthcare professional will help determine the right fluid intake for your specific condition.

Stress Management

Chronic kidney disease can be emotionally challenging. Implementing stress-reducing techniques such as mindfulness meditation, deep breathing exercises, and engaging in hobbies can have a positive impact on overall well-being. Seeking support from friends, family, or a support group can also provide valuable emotional support.

How to Monitor Your Kidney Health

Regular monitoring of kidney function is crucial in managing kidney disease and preventing further complications. This involves a combination of medical tests and lifestyle adjustments.

Blood Pressure Management

Controlling blood pressure is paramount in preserving kidney function. Regular blood pressure checks, both at home and during medical appointments, provide valuable information about your cardiovascular health. Medications, if prescribed, should be taken as directed to maintain optimal blood pressure levels.

Blood Tests
Blood tests, including serum creatinine, blood urea nitrogen (BUN), and estimated glomerular filtration rate (eGFR), provide critical information about kidney function. These tests should be conducted at regular intervals as recommended by your healthcare provider. Changes in these markers may indicate the need for adjustments in treatment or lifestyle.

Urine Tests
Urine tests, specifically for proteinuria and hematuria, can detect abnormalities in kidney function. Monitoring protein levels in the urine is essential in assessing the progression of kidney disease. Any significant changes should be reported to your healthcare team promptly.

Imaging Studies
In some cases, imaging studies like ultrasounds or CT scans may be conducted to assess the structure and size of the kidneys. These tests can help identify any physical abnormalities or blockages that may be impacting kidney function.

Regular Follow-Ups
Consistent follow-up appointments with your healthcare team are essential in managing kidney disease. These appointments allow for ongoing assessment, adjustments to treatment plans, and the opportunity to address any concerns or questions you may have.
In conclusion, effectively managing kidney disease requires a comprehensive approach that encompasses medication

management, lifestyle adjustments, and regular monitoring of kidney function. By working closely with your healthcare team and adopting positive lifestyle changes, you can take proactive steps towards maintaining optimal kidney health and overall well-being. Remember, every individual's journey with kidney disease is unique, and personalized care is key to achieving the best possible outcomes.

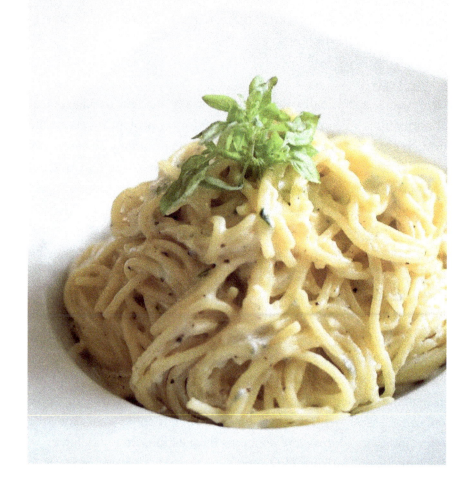

Tips for Staying Healthy and Active

In the pursuit of a healthy and fulfilling life with kidney disease, adopting a holistic approach that encompasses both physical and mental well-being is paramount. In this chapter, we will delve into essential tips for staying healthy and active, focusing on managing stress, getting adequate sleep, and avoiding the detrimental effects of alcohol and tobacco.

Managing Stress

Stress is a powerful force that can impact both mental and physical health. For individuals managing kidney disease, effectively coping with stress is crucial for overall well-being. Here are practical strategies to navigate and mitigate stress in your life.

Mindfulness Meditation

Engaging in mindfulness meditation is a potent tool in reducing stress levels. This practice involves bringing one's attention to the present moment, fostering a sense of calm and tranquility. Through guided meditation sessions or mindfulness apps, individuals can learn techniques to alleviate stress and promote mental clarity.

Deep Breathing Exercises

Conscious breathing exercises serve as an immediate antidote to stress. By taking slow, deep breaths, individuals activate the body's relaxation response, calming the nervous system. Simple practices like diaphragmatic breathing or progressive muscle relaxation can be easily incorporated into daily routines.

Engaging in Creative Outlets
Creative expression, whether through art, writing, or music, provides an avenue for emotional release and self-discovery. Engaging in these outlets offers a therapeutic means to process emotions, reduce stress, and cultivate a sense of accomplishment.

Physical Activity and Exercise
Regular physical activity is a potent stress-busting tool. Exercise prompts the release of endorphins, which are natural mood boosters. Activities like walking, yoga, or gentle stretching can be particularly beneficial for individuals with kidney disease. Consult with a healthcare provider to determine the appropriate level of exercise for your specific condition.

Seeking Emotional Support
Sharing your thoughts and feelings with trusted friends, family members, or support groups can provide invaluable emotional support. Additionally, seeking the guidance of a mental health professional, such as a counselor or therapist, can offer tailored strategies for managing stress.

Getting Enough Sleep
Quality sleep is a cornerstone of overall health, particularly for individuals managing kidney disease. Adequate rest supports immune function, cognitive health, and emotional well-being. Implementing good sleep hygiene practices can significantly enhance the quality of your sleep.

Establishing a Consistent Sleep Schedule
Maintaining a regular sleep routine helps regulate your body's internal clock. Aim to go to bed and wake up at the same time each day, even on weekends. Consistency reinforces your body's natural circadian rhythm.

Creating a Relaxing Bedtime Routine
Engaging in calming activities before bedtime signals your body that it's time to wind down. This may include activities like reading, gentle stretching, or practicing relaxation techniques. Avoid stimulating activities, such as intense exercise or screen time, in the hour leading up to sleep.

Designing a Comfortable Sleep Environment
Your sleep environment plays a significant role in the quality of your rest. Ensure your bedroom is conducive to sleep by maintaining a comfortable room temperature, using comfortable bedding, and minimizing light and noise disturbances. Consider investing in a supportive mattress and pillows.

Limiting Caffeine and Nicotine Intake
Caffeine and nicotine are stimulants that can disrupt your ability to fall asleep. Avoid consuming these substances in the hours leading up to bedtime. Instead, opt for decaffeinated beverages and consider implementing relaxation techniques to unwind.

Managing Pain and Discomfort
For individuals with kidney disease, managing any associated pain or discomfort is essential for restful sleep. Discuss pain management strategies with your healthcare provider to ensure you're receiving the appropriate support.

Avoiding Alcohol and Tobacco

Steering clear of alcohol and tobacco is pivotal for safeguarding kidney health and overall well-being. Both substances can have detrimental effects on the kidneys and exacerbate existing kidney conditions.

Alcohol Consumption

Alcohol places additional strain on the kidneys, as they are responsible for metabolizing and eliminating alcohol from the body. Excessive alcohol intake can lead to dehydration and high blood pressure, both of which are detrimental to kidney function. If you choose to consume alcohol, do so in moderation and consult with your healthcare provider for personalized guidance.

Tobacco Use

Tobacco use, in any form, is highly detrimental to kidney health. Smoking narrows blood vessels and reduces blood flow to the kidneys, impairing their ability to function optimally. Additionally, tobacco use increases the risk of high blood pressure and cardiovascular disease, further compromising kidney health. Seeking support to quit smoking is a crucial step in preserving kidney function.

Seeking Professional Guidance

If you're struggling with alcohol or tobacco dependence, seeking professional help is instrumental. Healthcare providers, counselors, and support groups can offer tailored strategies and resources to facilitate a successful journey toward sobriety and tobacco cessation.

In conclusion, adopting a proactive approach to managing stress, prioritizing quality sleep, and abstaining from alcohol and tobacco are integral components of a comprehensive kidney health regimen. By incorporating these practices into your daily life, you are taking significant strides toward safeguarding your kidney function and enhancing your overall well-being. Remember, small, consistent steps can lead to profound improvements in your health and quality of life.

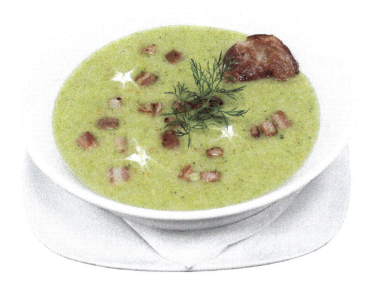

Foods to Avoid for Kidney Health

Maintaining a kidney-friendly diet is paramount for individuals with kidney disease. Certain foods can place additional stress on the kidneys or contribute to imbalances in vital nutrients. In this chapter, we will provide an extensive list of foods to avoid to promote optimal kidney health.

High-Sodium Foods
Excessive sodium intake can lead to fluid retention and elevated blood pressure, both of which are detrimental to kidney function. Avoid or limit the following high-sodium foods:

1. Processed and Canned Foods
2. Salted Snacks (Chips, Pretzels)
3. Deli Meats (Ham, Salami)
4. Canned Soups and Broths
5. Fast Food and Takeout
6. Pickled Vegetables
7. Soy Sauce and Other High-Sodium Condiments

High-Potassium Foods
For individuals with kidney disease, impaired potassium regulation can be a concern. Avoid or moderate intake of high-potassium foods to prevent potential complications:

8. Bananas

9. Oranges and Orange Juice
10. Potatoes (Especially Sweet Potatoes)
11. Tomatoes and Tomato Products (Sauce, Paste)
12. Avocados
13. Spinach and Kale
14. Beans and Lentils
15. Nuts and Seeds

High-Phosphorus Foods
Elevated phosphorus levels in the blood can lead to bone and heart complications. Individuals with kidney disease should be mindful of their phosphorus intake. Avoid or limit:

16. Dairy Products (Milk, Cheese, Yogurt)
17. Processed Meats (Hot Dogs, Sausages)
18. Organ Meats (Liver, Kidneys)
19. Colas and Dark Soft Drinks
20. Processed Baked Goods (Pastries, Doughnuts)

High-Protein Foods
While protein is essential for overall health, excessive protein intake can put strain on the kidneys. Moderation is key. Be cautious with:

21. Red and Processed Meats
22. Poultry with Skin
23. Fish with High Mercury Content (Shark, Swordfish)
24. Dairy Products with High Protein Content

Foods High in Oxalates
Oxalates can contribute to the formation of kidney stones in susceptible individuals. Limit consumption of foods high in oxalates:

25. Beets
26. Chocolate
27. Tea (Black and Green)
28. Nuts (Almonds, Cashews)
29. Rhubarb

Foods with Added Sugars

Excess sugar intake can lead to weight gain and metabolic complications, which can further impact kidney health. Avoid or limit foods with added sugars, including:

30. Sugary Drinks (Sodas, Fruit Juices)
31. Candies and Sweets
32. Processed Desserts (Cakes, Cookies)
33. Sweetened Cereals

Foods with High Phosphates

Phosphates found in processed foods can be challenging for individuals with kidney disease to metabolize. Avoid or limit:

34. Processed Cheese
35. Packaged Meats and Poultry
36. Fast Food Items (Burgers, Fries)
37. Packaged Snack Foods

Foods with Artificial Additives

Artificial additives, such as certain preservatives and colorings, can strain the kidneys. Avoid or limit foods with excessive additives:

38. Processed and Prepackaged Foods with Lengthy Ingredient Lists

39. Artificial Sweeteners (Aspartame, Saccharin)
40. Foods with Artificial Colorings and Flavorings

Excessive Fluids
While hydration is crucial, individuals with kidney disease may need to monitor fluid intake more closely. Avoid excessive fluid intake, especially if advised by your healthcare provider.

41. Large Amounts of Watermelon and Cucumbers
42. Drinking Excessive Amounts of Water in a Short Period

Alcohol and Tobacco
Alcohol and tobacco can have detrimental effects on kidney health. It is strongly advised to avoid or abstain from:

43. Excessive Alcohol Consumption
44. Smoking and Tobacco Use in Any Form

By being mindful of these foods to avoid and making conscious dietary choices, individuals with kidney disease can play an active role in maintaining optimal kidney function and overall well-being. Always consult with a healthcare professional or registered dietitian for personalized dietary recommendations tailored to your specific condition. Remember, small changes in your diet can lead to significant improvements in your kidney health and quality of life.